FITNESS AND HEALTH

Better weight maintenance; Increased energy levels; Lower odds of developing a metabolic disease

SHITTU DANIEL

TABLE OF CONTENT

Introduction

In the heart of a bustling city, Sarah found herself engulfed in the chaos of daily life. Amidst deadlines and responsibilities, her health took a backseat. Until one day, a wake-up call came in the form of exhaustion and aching muscles.

Determined to reclaim her vitality, she embarked on a journey to prioritize fitness and health. It wasn't easy; there were moments of doubt and setbacks. But with each step forward, she felt stronger and more alive. She discovered the joy of movement, the nourishment of wholesome foods, and the power of self-care.

As her body transformed, so did her mindset. No longer a burden, fitness became her sanctuary, a refuge from life's stresses. And as Sarah flourished, she became a beacon of inspiration to those around her, proving that investing in one's health is the greatest gift one can give to themselves.

Chapter 1

Basic

Making sure kids get the health benefits of exercise from an early age helps them value exercise as they get older. In addition, it's crucial to be active if you want to keep a healthy weight. Children who do not engage in sports or other physical activities have a higher risk of gaining weight as a result of sedentary activities like playing video games, watching television, and using the internet for extended periods of time. It may increase obesity risk by activity. In order to prevent youngsters from engaging in unhealthy behaviors, I advised that exercise be introduced to them as early as possible. It's crucial to select the physical activity that is best for you if you want a healthier body. Consequently, you must be aware of the best forms of exercise.

Boosting the intensity of your workout will bring you more rewards. Research suggests those who exercise regularly and for long periods may be likely to experience more health benefits than those who exercise less.

On the other hand, in our effort to lose weight we sometimes skip our meals to speed up the weight losing process. However, by doing this we are sacrificing our health. We don't need to do that. We just need to understand that losing weight is just a matter of burning enough calories that we consumed through our activities. Thus, starting a good physical exercise can well take care of that.

Chapter 2

Basics Of Physical Health

The act of reading this article indicates that you are physically ready to be healthy. What makes all these things about staying healthy so hard is the commitment you make to yourself.

Create Physical Health

Most of us would like to stay healthy, but not everyone can lead a healthy life. For this reason, many self-help tools have been developed to help you continue and ultimately reach your health goals, including this article.

To continue this seemingly difficult task, we must perceive it as something we do without question. We do these things because we believe they are essential and we can't go a day without doing them. The same concept applies if you choose to exercise every day increases. We must ensure having the attitude that exercise is the missing element to complete the physical fitness process, without which other efforts are not sufficient.

Learning the basics of physical health can help you understand what you are trying to achieve and how it can help you. First, there are four major elements of physical health.

1. **Cardiovascular Endurance** – These can be possible with activities such as swimming and running. Improving this component improves the delivery of oxygen and nutrients to body tissues while removing the waste products that have accumulated in the body.

2. **Strength** - These can be improved with a variety of weightlifting and stretching exercises. Improving this component would help them have a stronger muscle that allow them to react with less effort.

3. **Muscular endurance** – can be improved by doing push-ups every day, as it can effectively strengthen the muscles of the arms and shoulders. Improving this component improves the muscle's ability to withstand repeated contractions.

4. **Flexibility** - You can improve the extensibility of your muscles, which can be improved with regular stretching. Improving this component will improve your body's ability to move your joints and make the most of your muscles.

5. With these basics in mind, he recommends including activities that address the four elements in your exercise program so you can achieve optimal results. As a general guide, start your workout with a good warm-up and end with a gentle cool-down. Also, avoid overloading your body and avoiding strenuous exercise throughout the week.

Chapter 3

Basics of proper nutrition

Proper nutrition means providing the right amount and type of food your body needs to survive each day. Eating nutritious foods can help your body absorb the energy it needs and provide you with more consistent energy and mood throughout the day

Healthy Food

You can plan healthy and delicious meals as you go about your daily life. You don't have to starve to death to be ideally thin. Achieving a balanced and healthy mind and body requires a proper diet and regular exercise. Moderation is key. In all cases, whether in health or career, strong decision-making always plays a key role. Once you've decided and committed to staying healthy and eating right, you can definitely achieve it. If you believe you can achieve and maintain a balanced diet, you will. Take it step by step so you don't feel obligated. When you're happy with what you're doing, things become easier and you eventually become part of the system.

The goal of healthy eating is to maintain a healthy diet that can be maintained for a lifetime. So, once you know what foods are best for your health, set a standard, moderate diet.

Remember that your goals are long-term and not just reach your ideal weight. , just make sure you're getting the right balance of minerals.

On the other hand, when you eat, you take your time and grind your food. Not only will you enjoy your meal, but it will improve your digestion. Stop eating even if you think you've had enough! It usually takes some time for the brain to receive the signal that the stomach is already full. Fruits and vegetables are rich in antioxidants, fiber, vitamins, and minerals, and contain fewer calories in the body, so consuming fruits and vegetables at every meal can help complete a healthy diet. Colored fruits and vegetables are more concentrated in vitamins and minerals and can provide more benefits. Eating 5 pieces a day is enough. Also, eat enough healthy carbs and avoid unhealthy fats. Whole grains are the best source of healthy carbs that can provide you with sustained energy throughout the day. It's also high in antioxidants and phytochemicals, which help prevent cancer, coronary artery disease, and diabetes. On the other hand, eating healthy fats helps nourish your cells, brain, heart, hair, nails, and skin also helps.

Chapter 4

Exercise Basics

Most of us know how important exercise is in our daily lives. It's one of the backbones of our overall health. Additionally, exercise is effective in reducing stress and emotional setbacks. If you exercise regularly, you're more likely to stay healthier, happier, and calmer most of the time than someone who doesn't exercise as much.

Keep Fit

Despite knowing how important exercise is, we still can't find the time to exercise and stick to a regular exercise schedule. Why should we exercise in the first place? What do you have for us? Learn more about exercise concepts and benefits. Regular exercise has countless benefits, but here are the main ones:

1. An effective way to lose weight while staying healthy and slim as you age

2. Effective in maintaining bone mass.

3. Lowers bad cholesterol, blood sugar and blood pressure

4. Effective for relieving stress and improving sleep

5 Maintain good cardiovascular health, energy, flexibility, and good looks.

Above are the most well-known benefits of exercise. Many people feel that they are already exercising in regular activities such as gardening, cleaning, washing the car or washing the dishes, and expect to get the same benefits of structured exercise. Unfortunately, daily activity is not the same as structured exercise, where you can expect great results. Your daily activity will only help you burn calories and stay active. So, if you want to get the best results, you should do both regularly.

To get off to a good start, consult your doctor for advice as there may be some restrictions on your exercise. However, most of the exercises are safe to perform. Restrictions apply only to people suffering from chronic diseases, heart problems, arthritis, bone problems, high blood pressure, respiratory problems, etc.

Once you've taken the first steps, find the exercise that works best for you and make it a routine. Please do not strain yourself. Gradually but regularly. Try to enjoy what you are doing If you don't do this, you will soon become discouraged. You can change your routine and try other fitness exercises as long as it works for you. This should be done to reduce boredom in the long run.

Chapter 5

Basics of Mental Disorders

A mental disorder is defined as a condition that affects how a person feels, thinks and acts, with or without the influence of those around them. People with mental disorders may show signs of mild to severe mental retardation, depending on the person's condition. Most patients find it difficult to cope with even the simplest routines and demands at work and at home.

Develop A Healthy Mind

There is no exact cause of mental illness. However, research shows that mental illness is caused by any of the following factors, or a combination of psychological, biological, genetic, and environmental problems, and is not really a personal weakness. Therefore, in most cases, the condition does not seem to require medical or pharmaceutical intervention and cannot be relieved by simple self-discipline.

After the cause is the nature of the mental illness. Mental illness can be effectively treated with the right approach. Therefore, knowing its type can help improve the recovery process. Below are the most common types of mental disorders. Psychotic disorders - are described as distorted patterns of thought and consciousness. The most common symptom is hallucinations. People with psychotic disorders may experience strange sights and sounds that they perceive as real events, despite clear ideas of delusions. A well-known example of a psychotic disorder is schizophrenia. is.

Personality Disorders – These disorders are characterized by an extremely dogmatic personality that makes the individual or those around them feel stressed or upset. This is why people with personality disorders continue to encounter problems at work, school, home, and even in their personal and social relationships with others. It's from Examples of this condition include obsessive-compulsive personality disorder, paranoid personality disorder, and antisocial personality disorder.

Mood disorders - These disorders are also known as mood disorders. They have been described as having an unrelenting sense of sadness or euphoria, or fluctuations in the two extremes. For example, a very happy state is a very sad state. Examples of this disorder are bipolar disorder and depression.

Anxiety Disorders – People with anxiety disorders react to certain situations with great fear, resulting in extreme nervousness, sweating, and rapid heartbeat. Including but not limited to anxiety disorders, and social anxiety disorders.

Addictive Disorders - These are characterized by an uncontrollable urge to do things that are harmful to oneself and others. Examples include theft, gambling, alcohol, and drug addiction.

Eating Disorders - These disorders are characterized by extreme attitudes, emotions, and behaviors related to food and weight. Examples include bulimia nervosa, binge eating disorder, and anorexia nervosa.

Chapter 6

Basics Of Stress

Stress is defined as a reaction to something that takes a toll on us physically, mentally and emotionally, thereby affecting our balance. When stressful events occur, the fight or flight response is triggered, causing adrenaline and cortisol to spike in the body to keep you awake and alive.

Relax!

Less stress is good, but maintaining it over the long term can have a big impact on your overall health. Stress is inevitable, but the best way to prevent it from lasting long is to change your response to stress. how are you going to do this?

We need to understand the stress and why it needs to be present in our lives. There are multiple types and levels of stress. So it makes sense that we are affected in many ways. To deal with stress effectively, you must first understand the type of stress you are experiencing. This way, you can tune your mind and body to release stress as quickly as possible.

Stress can be both good and bad in your life, so stress shouldn't always be perceived as a bad thing. Stress gets worse the longer it stays in us. The good thing about moderate stress is that it gives us energy. If you can distinguish between good and bad strains, you can use them to your advantage. Our health can be severely affected by stress if we take it for granted. Sometimes I get sick. In addition, 'chronic stress' can also affect mental health and lead to emotional instability. Before that happens, you have to stop the madness before it completely ruins you.

Studies have also shown that stress affects the body. This is because once you experience stress overload, you are less likely to take care of yourself. You pay less attention to your appearance, or worse, care less about your eating habits and the types of foods you eat, which can change the way your body processes food. It has a big impact.

Stress can also affect our lifestyles and relationships. When you're stressed, you feel like you don't have enough time to fulfill your responsibilities. The result is less participation and rarely seeing friends and family. Because stress can make someone grumpy, it can also hurt loved ones because of unpredictable moods.

Chapter 7

Mental Health Basics

In general, it takes a sound mind to do things right. Our mental powers help us to be effective in what we do. Also, keeping order plays an important role in our lives. Mental health is a general term. However, it refers to our general state of mind with a high level of mental health and the absence of mental disorders. happy heart, happy life

A person's ability to stay happy and enjoy life can also be measured by mental health. This is because our mental faculties greatly influence our emotions, and how we express and react. Poor mental health impairs judgment because the mind does not function rationally. Mental illness changes the way you see and react to life. Most of the time you are emotionally unstable. This makes many people without healthy mental health vulnerable targets for depression and other mental disorders. Our mental health can be affected by many factors, including physical condition, environment, work, relationships, and genetics. Today, much research has been deliberately done to give high priority and importance to the question of how people achieve mental health. and creative life.

In general, areas of our lives that can be greatly affected by our mental state are our spirituality, work, relationships, emotions, relaxation, and self-determination. We must understand that being emotionally healthy does not mean that we are not free from uncontrollable and unexpected problems. But a healthy mind and spirit will help you face any challenge with a better perspective and help you stay focused, flexible, and results-oriented. To maintain good mental health, we must prevent all risk factors that can lead to mental and emotional instability. When faced with a difficult situation, focus on identifying the root cause of the problem and knowing exactly how to deal with it.

Finally, we all want to live a beautiful and peaceful life, so we should fill our lives with relaxed, positive people and always choose constructive relationships instead of the opposite.

Chapter 8
Basics of Spiritual Health

Our minds are not technically part of our physical attributes but are considered an integral part of our human wholeness. Our bodies function in harmony with our minds and soul. So, each of them can affect the other. However, if you care about your physical and mental health, you should also care about your mental health.

Many of us do not realize that the body can heal faster because a healthy mind can provide good energy while it is in the healing process. It is considered part of the treatment because it is very helpful in managing the pain and complications associated with Mental health can be achieved when your life is in perfect harmony. It means finding peace in times of distress and hope in times of despair. Life is completely different when the mind is healthy. When you have a serious illness, you can forget your beliefs, feel like the illness is eating you away, and leave your beliefs alone. But what we don't know is that when we are sane, we have the power to fight all sorts of diseases simply because we are perfect beings. So when our body, mind, and spirit are in harmony, we have a better chance of a speedy recovery.

On the other hand, if you feel that your mental health is not good, take some time to reflect and see how you are living your life from a wider perspective. Listen to and feel the stillness. In this way, you can better understand the essence of your life, what makes you feel complete, and exactly where you find your inner strength. Above all, keep a positive outlook on life.

Chapter 9

Benefits For Maintaining Overall Health

Maintaining overall good health offers several long-term benefits. Regular exercise helps children develop strong bones, healthy joints, and muscles. Even into adulthood, consistent exercise can help shed excess fat and make way for a leaner physique. In addition, the risk of diabetes, bone fractures, heart disease, especially colon cancer, and other serious illnesses. reduce the Studies also show that exercise can help reduce stress and depression by about 50%, with immediate results. good stuff

Another way to maintain overall health is to combine regular exercise with supplements. Because today, due to the high demands in our personal and professional lives, it is very difficult for each of us to have a truly balanced diet.

Dietary supplements can meet the necessary nutrients our bodies need even when we are unable to get the balanced nutritional intake we want. We have become more aware of the benefits of wellness products that contain food. Therefore, it is easier for us to choose the nutritional supplement that best suits our needs. Most nutritional supplements on the market today contain herbs, vitamins, minerals and amino acids. considered to be a substance.

In addition to the general benefits of supplements, there are other attendant benefits that specific supplements can provide.

For pregnant women, folic acid intake significantly reduces the chances of having a child with spina bifida. Niacin produces good cholesterol, as does omega-3 fatty acids, which lower triglyceride levels. In ancient times, people discovered several plants and herbs that helped them stay physically and mentally healthy. For this reason, even though modern people no longer eat natural, nutritious foods, modern scientists are working more We have done a lot of research and developed herbs and dietary supplements.

Wrap Up

Ultimately, you need to stick to a routine that enriches your physical health, combined with a balanced diet, the supplements your body and mind need, and your efforts to manage your overall health. You'll feel more confident knowing you're taking essential steps to improve your overall health. Enjoy life at a happier pace and learn to relax. You can use the steps you just learned to get your mind and body in top shape and live a peaceful life. I wish you good luck!

www.ingramcontent.com/pod-product-compliance
Lightning Source LLC
Chambersburg PA
CBHW072346270726
48659CB00023B/2401